Aging Backwards

Prevent Premature Aging and Look 10 Years Younger!

AGING BACKWARDS
Prevent Premature Aging and Look 10 Years Younger!
How To Stay Young and Healthy After Menopause

Dominique Kaneza

Table of Contens

Introduction

Do not get desperate if you just entered your menopause age. In fact, you should be more cheerful than ever. From the latest WHO report, we know that even though there is a rapid decrease in our hormonal functions, we can still enjoy our youthful, healthy, and happy life after our menopause. Menopause is a good beginning for a healthier and more vibrant life than ever. It helps us to overcome the next part of our life as adult women.

As we get older, our cells degenerate and we begin to lose some of our body functions one by one. Menopause is just one of the symptoms. However, with a healthy lifestyle, we might be able to prevent our body from degenerating too rapidly. You can still have an idea life with a simple understanding of how your body works. There is no need to perform cosmetic surgery to grab your beautiful youth back, if only you know the natural ways to preserve your beauty. In this book, you will learn many ways to stay young & healthy and to uncover your natural beauty.

There are four key elements in staying young and healthy after your menopause: *physical exercises, mind exercises, healthy diet,* and *rest.* You will learn each of these key elements in this book. Pay close attention to each of them as they will teach you how easy it is to grab the youth back, but only if you have the commitment to do so.

Causes of Premature Aging

It is always interesting to discuss about women's worst nightmare: aging. As we always try to look beautiful, we also deal with the fact that sometimes our skin does not share the same idea. Since then facial exercises and cosmetic products have become our 'best friend'in every day life. However, do we truly understand what causes skin aging, especially premature aging? Let us find them out.

1. Sun exposure

   Getting that warm feeling on your face skin is so tempting, but do not trick yourself. This tempting warm sensation is a particular sign that your facial skin is starting to wrinkle. Therefore, next time you are planning to get that sunshine, do not forget to bring along your sunscreen.

2. Facial expressions

   Every time we feel sad, angry, or anything out of happiness, we usually express them on our faces, but that is not the only thing we do. We move our skin muscles to create that expression and show everyone our feelings. However, we do not realize that when we move those muscles we have triggered our cells to wrinkle. Yes, that sounds worse than we think. Therefore, next time I think you know what expressions to choose: happiness or sadness.

3. Smoking

Smoking is toxic. Not only can it ruin your body, but also your beauty. This dirty little habit will make you look much older than your present age. You should quit this habit if you want to preserve your beauty and stay healthy after your menopause. Yes, it is difficult at first, but as long as you keep that intention in your mind, you will always find the strength to fight it.

4. Stress

Women are so eager to react to stress and sometimes, we believe it is impossible to get rid of stress from our life. However, as we learned from making happy expressions on our face, living without stress should relieve our muscles from creating skin wrinkles. So, relax a bit and think about something funny. This will help eliminate stress. It is good for your beauty, charisma, and life though.

5. Lack of Sleep

Our body needs to rest after the whole daylong. While we rest, our cells regenerate and fix any broken part of our body, including our wrinkles. Therefore, in other words, if we do not get enough sleep, our body will not get enough time to fix those wrinkles. It means, instead of eliminating those wrinkles, they will stay for quite a long time on your face and even get worse than before. However, getting too much sleep is also not good as our body functions will degenerate faster than ever.

6. Alcohol

Several factors create wrinkles. One of them is hormonal balance in our skin. Keeping the balance is a good thing to keep the wrinkles off our face, but drinking alcohol is certainly not the recommended advice you could get in getting those wrinkles off. It is because alcohol creates not only hormonal imbalance, but also degenerative functions of our body. In the other words, the more you drink alcohol, the more you destroy your body, create wrinkles, and lose your beauty.

7. Lack of Moisture

There is a saying that a woman is as beautiful as an angel. We are the creature of the beauty itself. While we always do our best to look beautiful, there is one fact we cannot avoid: our skin needs water to stay tight, smooth, and fascinating. Without enough water, we should deal with one of the worst nightmare of all women: dry skin. It 'invites' the three worst skin nightmare: wrinkle, bleed, and crack. Giving enough moisturizer to you skin is the simplest way to avoid these nightmares, but remember not to give it too much as there would be too much water in your skin, leading to the wrinkles worse than if you have dry skin.

Exercise to Avoid Premature Aging

As we get older, we face higher risk of premature aging. As women, we constantly dream about how to stop the clock and make our beauty last forever. Unfortunately, none of us has that gift. The only power we have in our hands is the power to use all available resources inside and outside our body to slow the clock. We may get older, but no one will realize that with that age, we still have a perfect, healthy, and happy life as young women have. All these dreams are possible with the following exercises you can use to slow the clock and preserve your beauty:

1. Endurance training

    Endurance training helps your body to improve its cardiovascular function, including but not limited to keeping your heart muscle supple, arteries flexible, optimizing heart's ability for oxygen distribution, lowering your resting heart rate, and reducing the risk of high blood pressure.

    Endurance training is also accountable for protecting your body metabolism from premature aging. It ensures our skin to always getting all the nutrients it needs to stay beautiful and healthy. It keeps the excess fat away, increases the response of our body tissues to Insulin, and delivers oxygen, water, and other nutrients to our skin.

With endurance training, you can improve your sleep and boost your mood. You will be able to counter stress, depression, and anxiety. In other words, you can keep your muscles from creating those wrinkles. In order to prevent premature aging, you need to exercise regularly. You need to gradually build your exercise up to 3 – 4 hours per week.

Recommended endurance training includes walking, biking, jogging, racquet sports, swimming, cross-country skiing, rowing, playing golf, and doing aerobic dance.

2. Resistance exercises

Resistance exercises focus on keeping your muscles healthy and preserving your bone calcium. In order to prevent premature aging, resistance exercises can help build up your muscle mass, supplying it with enough water and nutrients, leading to less wrinkles and any unwanted appearance on your skin. You can simply use resistance bands to do the workout.

3. Flexibility exercises

Flexibility exercises will help you fight premature aging by keeping your body supple. An ideal workout requires approximately 20 minutes of exercise, which you should repeat 2 – 3 times a week. Simple exercises such as stretching exercises should also be able to help you warm up your muscles before the exercises and cool them down after the exercises. If you love doing Yoga, it will also do the job.

4. Exercises for balance

Balance exercises will help you counter some common effects of premature aging by lowering the risk of falls, avoiding injuries, engaging various muscle groups, and fix muscle problems. I recommend taking these exercises 4 – 5 times a week with barefoot and three moves each.

Here are my three favorite balance exercises:

a. Stork swim

1. Using your left foot as support, bend your right knee, then raise this knee behind you until it reaches your hip level

2. With your palms up, reach your hands straight out

3. Focus on your right leg, bend it forward, then extend it straight behind you.

4. Hold for 8 – 10 seconds.

5. Return to the initial position

6. Do 20 – 25 reps.

7. Switch to your left knee and repeat the whole steps while keeping your arms straight.

b. T-slide

   1. Keep your feet together, then lift your heels and balance only on your toes

   2. Reach your left and right hands to both your sides and keep the palms facing forward

   3. Use your arms to pulse 1 inch both backward and forward. Do 25 reps

   4. Now, face your palms toward your house ceiling. Do this for 25 reps

   5. Then, face your palms backward. Do this for 25 reps.

c. Russian twist

   1. Use the floor as your mattress, sit and bend your knees. Then cross your left foot under the another one at the ankle

   2. Now touch your knees with both your hands, and then lift your feet. Next, you need to lean back 45 degrees

   3. Loosely clasp your hands in front of you, and then lower your right elbow and the left one towards the mattress. Do this for 25 reps.

   4. Switch sides and do for 25 reps.

How to Keep the Body Biologically Young

*Through perseverance many people win
success out of what seemed destined to
be certain failure.*

--Benjamin Disraeli

For each day we pass, our body loses around 430 billion cells. Even though our body can quickly replace these cells, the number of cells we lose in every single day is quite large. With premature aging, the number might even get higher than 430 billion. Regenerating broken and dead cells is the natural way for our body to stay young and healthy. This is how exactly we can live the life as we expect. However, without proper steps, our body might just lose its ability to regenerate its cells and fasten the premature aging.

The key lies on this question. How can we keep our body biologically young?

1.   Take a break

When you experience stress, your body releases adrenaline and cortisol hormone. Both these hormones are responsible for increasing heartbeat and blood pressure, which in turn are responsible for triggering and accelerating premature aging.

Here is how you can fight it:

For 10 – 20 minutes a day (1-2 exercises), try to sit in your favorite, quite place. Then, close your eyes, breathe, and relax. Roll your shoulders, neck, and head. On each exhale, repeat the special phrase you can pick by our own, such as "Thank you." When you are at the end of each exercise, spare a few minutes to close your eyes and allow every thoughts in the day to flow slowly into your mind. That is it.

2.   Consume Omega 3

Omega-3 fatty acids can prevent signs of premature aging, especially the visible ones, by reducing your body inflammation. Other benefits include mood stabilizer, maintaining bone strength and improving enzymes ability to distribute body fat evenly.

Per medical recommendation, your Omega-3 intake should come from natural sources, such as wild salmon (6.9 grams of Omega 3 from 3-ounce serving) or walnuts (9.2 grams of Omega-3 from a 1.5-ounce serving)

3.   Exercise regularly

In its last report, the US National Institute on Aging revealed that regular exercises have diverse benefits, such as toning muscles, losing weight, building healthy bones, and boosting mood. However, they are not the only benefits you can get if you exercise regularly. By walking, swimming, or jogging 20 minutes a day for 3 times a week, you can also reduce your anxiety and stress, which is important, if you want to keep your body biologically young.

4.   Experience love

If you want to keep your body biologically young and live a happy life, make sure you put love at the central part of your life. Not only it can help your body to reduce stress, but also improve your self-esteem. In fact, by experiencing love, your body will get enough trigger to improve your cardiovascular health and boost your immune system.

Well, I think I should leave this part to you on how to experience love. Am I right?

5.   Do Yoga

While improved flexibility, reduced stress, better posture, improved mood, and better energy have become the most common benefits of doing Yoga, Yoga is also quite popular for the benefits of doing its Yogic breathing. This mind-body breathing technique can help you in oxygenating your cells, eliminating free radicals and toxins from your body, improving your immune system, and preserving your everlasting beauty. These various benefits of doing Yoga simply come from the nature of Yoga itself that combine the works inside your body as well as outside it.

Here is how you can use Yoga to keep your body young:

Practice Yoga at least 3 times a week, at least 30 minutes each.

6.   Get some super fruits

There is a good reason people name some fruits as super fruits due to their ability not only to keep your body healthy, but also to keep it young.

Pomegranate is one of them. This super fruit can help you lower your blood pressure, cholesterol, prevent atherosclerosis, reduce the risk of suffering from Alzheimer, prevent and cure cancer, and protect your skin from UV damage.

Another promising fruit that can keep your body young is goji berry. Containing vitamin C 500 times higher than an orange, this super fruit is the house of various nutrients to keep your body young and healthy, including carotenoids, iron, 18 amino acids, zinc, magnesium, calcium, vitamin B1, B6, E, and E. This super fruit will keep your body young and healthy by improving your sleeping ability, reducing fat, improving your immune system, and improving your memory.

7.   Drink green tea

As we get older, our body function degenerates. Therefore, if you believe living a biologically young body also means living with high-functioning body, then you should consider inserting green tea into your diet. This specific tea can help you reduce the risk of various diseases, including breast cancer, bladder carcinoma, lung cancer, obesity, Alzheimer, and colorectal carcinoma.

To keep your body biologically young and healthy, drink atleast 2 – 3 cups of green tea daily.

8. Take skin supplements

Being young also means being beautiful with smooth and wrinkle-free skin. If you want to live as beautiful as a young woman does, then you should consider taking retinol. This vitamin A will help your skin to peel, allowing you to get your silky, rosy, and supple layer skin. In the other words, this vitamin A will help you in getting your beautiful skin back again, reducing the worry for the premature aging. It will help you in reducing any fine line, tightening your pores, and improving your skin texture.

9. Exercise mental aerobics

Being young also means having brain as sharp as young woman. If you want to prevent premature aging, then make sure you prevent your brain from suffering from cognitive declining.

Here is how you can exercise your mind and get the bright brain as young women have:

Strengthen your mind by playing Sudoku, Brain Games, or crossword puzzles. You can also try other games that uses sequences, words, or numbers to sharpen both spheres of your brain.

20 Easy Ways to Prevent Premature Aging

It always seems impossible until it's done.

--Nelson Mandela

Can we prevent premature aging? Women always ask this one problematic question in their life. The answer is obvious. Even though we do not possess the gift to stop the clock, we do have the access to all resources to slow down the time. It means we can do something to prevent the premature aging and live as healthy, happy, and beautiful as young woman. However, using these resources is the less intriguing question we should deal when it comes to preventing premature aging.

The biggest question lies on this matter: how much control do we have on preventing premature aging?

Our DNA contains the fate of our body and with age, it will degenerate. Our skin will wear and tear, our eyes will lose sight, our feet will lose strength to move, and many other things. However, our DNA also spare us some rooms where we can put our effort to slow down the process or prevent the premature aging. The following four points should be able to draw a line about things we can do to prevent premature aging.

Exercise Routines for Any Schedule

If you search the internet, there are many questions about the truth whether routine exercises can help fighting premature aging. This is a good question, which you should ask to yourself first. The fact is, even though the answer is obvious, yet there are still so many people questioning the truth.

Exercises can help you prevent premature aging, but it does not work like a charm. You cannot perform an exercise in a day and few hours later, you are no longer dealing with premature aging problem. Exercises does not work like that. Exercises prevent premature aging by optimizing your cell mitochondria. As you can see, each time we exercise, it triggers our cells to burn energy 'deposit' in our tissues. There are common energy deposits in our body: protein, carbohydrate, and fat. In order to transform these deposits into energy, we need an intracellular energy production unit we call as mitochondria. The more we exercise, the more active our mitochondria will be. With enough sleep and healthy diet, our cells will be able to produce enough energy, which is essential in the distribution of nutrients and oxygen to every part of our body. Without this energy, we will have increased risk of premature aging itself.

As we focus these exercises to prevent premature aging, there are somethings we should consider.

1. If you exercise outdoor, you must remember that outdoor exercises expose your skin to UV damage.

2. If you engage yourself in outdoor cardiovascular exercises, make sure you come with a healthy diet to supplement your training. Your diet must contain ascorbic acid, lipoid acid, and glutamine. You should take these supplements at least fifteen minutes before your exercise to reduce both the tissue inflammatory and oxidative damage.

3. If you choose to exercise in water, such as swimming, you must remember that there are certain chemical substances in water that may trigger hormonal imbalance in your skin. Therefore, it is necessary to wash your skin directly after the exercises to prevent any further damage. You can also use fragrance-free, chemical-free moisturizer as additional treatment to your skin.

4. The best thing to remember about exercises is hygiene. It is important to keep yourself, especially your skin clean before doing any exercise. By washing your skin before the exercise, you have prevented any harmful agents from sinking deeper through your skin pores during the exercise due to the rise in temperature. With your sweat covering your body, it is a perfect chance for the bacteria, viruses, and other harmful agents to ruin your body and accelerating the aging process, instead of preventing it from happening. With all the sacrifices you have made, I am certain this is exactly the thing you are not seeking forward.

5. Do not forget to hydrate yourself before, during, and after your exercises to prevent dehydration and 'additional' wrinkles. After everything you have done during the exercises, you certainly do not want to suffer from

dehydration or even get extra wrinkles just because you forget to drink enough water.

With these things in mind, there are some exercises, which I found useful in preventing premature aging. In order to reach the optimum result, I combine three key elements in preventing premature aging: mind, commitment, and body. The following exercises will help you understand how exactly this combination will help you to prevent premature aging and get your healthy life back:

1. Take minimum 5 minutes a day to perform a mindful meditation

    Preventing premature aging is not only about getting your desired physical state, but also a peaceful mind. You cannot live a healthy, happy life and even prevent premature aging if there is no connection between your mind and your body. Spending at least 5 minutes a day in a mindful meditation will help you in building bridge between your mind and body. Furthermore, it is only with a peaceful mind, which can strengthen you if there is anything that may block your way in preventing premature aging. If you like, you can add some relaxing music in your meditation to help you enter the deep, peaceful state of your mind. It will not take all of your time, but there is no doubt it can give something you can never expect to lose in your life.

2. Get yourself a self-massage after each workout to relax your nervous system as well as release any tension

Your muscles are not the only thing you train in each exercise you take. In fact, you also train your mind or your nervous system. Your muscles will certainly get tense during each workout, but please do not forget that your nervous system also bears the same load. Therefore, giving yourself a self-massage will help your nervous system to relax a bit after the workout. This is important, as I believe you are not expecting to have a not-so-peaceful mind even though you can prevent the premature aging. With your success in preventing premature aging, I believe you will not spare any time to mourn about your failure in having a healthy and relax nervous system.

3. You can also try some restorative activities to give your mind a peace, such as Yoga, book reading, walking, massages, swimming and other similar exercises

    Exercises to prevent premature aging does not always mean the physical ones. You can also take some restorative exercises to give your mind a peaceful state. If you love reading a book, then it would be great. By reading books, you train your mind to stay young and healthy in keeping memories, learning, and adopting. I would also like to recommend other exercises that may train your brain such as playing Sudoku, crossword puzzles, and any other similar brain games. It may not exercise your muscles, but they do train your brain to stay as sharp as young people have. As you may have heard, premature aging affects not only your body, but also your mind at the same time.

4. Be honest with yourself about your commitment to live a healthy and happy life as it will help you prevent premature aging.

    Another exercise can help you prevent premature aging. In fact, this exercise may exceed the importance of both physical and mind exercise. Before you step into both these exercise, you must exercise your commitment first. There is no chance you can prevent premature aging if you have a little or even no commitment at all. You might have spent the whole year to exercise your muscles, smooth your skin, and train your brain, but without a dedication in your heart and mind, all those exercises will be meaningless. Therefore, before any exercise, please be honest with yourself about how you would like to commit yourself to prevent premature aging. As your exercises progress, you will soon realize how this commitment exercise will help you prevent premature aging by strengthening and fortifying the premature lack of commitment to stay young and healthy.

Your Diet and Aging

There is an old saying: you are what you eat. Foods we eat not only determines our identity, but also our life. From our brain to our bones, our life depends on food we eat and beverages we drink. Therefore, if we question about how to prevent premature aging by living a healthy diet, then we should consider about food we should put on our plate and things we should keep from our plate.

a. Foods we should put on our plate

1. Colorful vegetables and fruits

Colorful fruits and vegetables come with high antioxidants level, which is a key element in preventing premature aging. So, make sure at each meal you take, you have filled at least half your place with these colorful vegetables and fruits, such as deep red tomatoes, carrots, leafy greens, and blueberries. Their antioxidant contents can help your body in keeping harmful molecules away from your healthy cells. For optimum result, you need to take at least five servings a day of these healthy meals.

Along with the antioxidants, colorful fruits and vegetables also come with high level of beta-carotene, zinc, and vitamin C. These nutrients will protect your eyes from macular degeneration which usually results in vision loss. If you are suffering from this disease, these foods may help you to slow the progress: collard, kale, mustard greens, spinach, cantaloupe, oranges, peppers, and corn.

Some specific antioxidants, like vitamin C, will also preserve your skin beauty, while another antioxidant we know as resveratrol is accountable for lowering the risk of premature aging, heart disease, and cancer. Both grapes and red wine are the common source of this antioxidant.

2. Whole grains

   Fiber-rich grains, such as barley, quinoa, brown rice, wheat, and oats can help you reduce the chances of developing type-2 diabetes as well as keeping your blood vessels healthy. For the optimum result, you need to take three servings a day.

3. Fish

   Omega-3 fatty acids in fish is your sword against premature aging. It helps you keep your heart healthy as well as reduce stroke and Alzheimer risk. Daily intake of two servings a week of tuna, lake trout, or salmon will provide the best impact to your health.

4. Dairy products

   Dairy products are rich in both fortified vitamin D and calcium. These nutrients are important to build your bone mass and keep osteoporosis away from your life. Daily intake of three cups of dairy products will keep both the vitamin D and calcium level adequate in your body. You can choose either yoghurt, low-fat milk, or other dairy products to put in your diet. Please remember to avoid taking regular dairy products as they are usually high in cholesterol. Taking low-fat dairy products instead of the regular ones will help reducing heart disease risk.

   In case you cannot consume or get dairy products; you can use cereals, almond milk, or soymilk with high level of vitamin D and calcium to substitute the dairy products.

5. Nuts

Nuts are one of the most popular sources of healthy fats. In fact, experts believe they are among the rarest sources. Taking nuts as your snack may help you lower high blood pressure and cholesterol risk up to 20%. This benefit simply exceeds the amount of daily intake you should take which is 0.25 ounce or approximately four almonds.

6. Lentils and beans

Our body needs protein to prevent premature aging by regenerating our cells and these foods are just the perfect source of plant-based proteins and fiber. Therefore, if you can't have red meat with saturated fat to prevent the premature aging, you can have beans and lentils instead. Other benefits include lowering the risk of both diabetes and heart disease.

b. Foods we should keep away from our plate

1. Foods with high saturated fats

Bakery treats, high-fat dairy products, and high-fat meat are the most common sources for saturated fats. Unless you lose your commitment to prevent premature aging, taking these foods may clog your arteries, resulting in heart problems. You surely do not want to take these foods.

2. Sugar

Sugar should become one of your biggest concerns in preventing premature aging. Taking too much sugar may bring tiny differences between your blood sugar levels and roller coaster riding downs and ups at high speed. Furthermore, excess calories due to the inadequate level of insulin may also result in insulin resistance. Insulin resistance is the common cause of type 2 diabetes. This disease is quite popular for damaging our blood vessels and increasing the risk of heart diseases. This is the reason there is a saying, "The less sugar we eat, the healthier our life will become." There is no doubt about the truth in this saying.

3. Salt

At the second place, with the similar impact like sugar, we have salt. Taking too much sodium or salt may result in increasing blood pressure. If you keep this lifestyle, your brain, eyes, and kidneys may suffer from long-term damage. However, without enough salt, you may also suffer from goiter and hypothyroidism. Per medical recommendation, the highest daily intake of sodium is 2,400 milligrams. This amount is equal with 1 teaspoon of table salt.

If you are suffering from high blood pressure, chronic kidney disease, or diabetes, you should reduce the amount to less than 1,500 mg of daily intake or approximately ½ teaspoon of table salt. Women after menopause should also carefully consider their salt daily intake. I strongly recommend limiting your daily intake up to 1,500 milligrams.

Most people, not only women, fail to realize the amount of salt they have taken when they consume too many boxed, frozen, or canned foods. These types of foods usually come with high sodium level. It is because salt is also a natural preserving agent. Food factories use salt to keep their foods last for weeks without adding artificial preservatives. Therefore, make sure you have checked the nutrition label before you purchase them. Your foods may not taste 'as delicious as they used to be,' but as long as to prevent premature aging, there is no such thing as bad as living a healthy diet. On top of that, as the time goes, you tongue will learn to adopt and you will get that delicious taste back again and now it comes without any complaint at all.

Natural Healings Methods

Premature aging is merely a major post-menopause syndrome, which occurs naturally at our 50. At the other side, menopause is actually a signal our body gives to show there is a hormonal imbalance inside our body, causing degenerative functions of our cells. There is no way we can stop it, but with certain remedies, we can slow the process and reduce the risk. I will always recommend you to take natural healing methods, as they contain no side effect for our body.

1. Olive oil

   With high level of minerals, natural fatty acids, and vitamins, olive oil can lighten your wrinkles, tighten sagging skin, and fine lines. Olive oil is also popular for being a powerful antioxidant. You can use this oil to hydrate your skin, maintain its suppleness, and preserve its elasticity.

   How to do it:

   a. Pour 2 – 3 drops of this oil on your palm

   b. Clean your face first and apply the oil gently on your clean neck and face, using circular motion

   c. Repeat the massage for 5 minutes before night rest; you can wash it off in the morning

2. Aloe Vera

   Aloe Vera is quite famous for being natural remedy for premature aging and other post-menopause systems, due to high malic acid it contains. Along with high zinc content, it increases the suppleness and elasticity of your skin by moisturizing it and improve the production of skin collagen.

How to do it:

a. Cut off an *Aloe Vera* leaf and scrape out its gel

b. Apply the gel on clean face

c. Softly massage your face for 8 minutes in circular motion.

d. Wait for 15 minutes and use lukewarm water to wash it off

3. Fenugreek

Fenugreek fights premature aging by using niacin and vitamin B3 to recover damaged skin cells and regenerate new tissues and cells. As the result, you will no longer have hyper pigmentation wrinkles, age spots, crow's feet, and fine lines at the corner of your lips, eyes, and forehead.

How to do it:

a. Take a handful of the seeds

b. Take a teaspoon of honey and add it to the seeds

c. Mix them well

d. Apply on your clean neck and face.

e. Wait for 1 hour before washing it off.

4.   Egg whites

With high level of riboflavin, magnesium, potassium, and proteins, egg whites can counter any side effect of menopause and premature aging. It helps repairing skin tissue. It also reduces the effects of oxidative stress and free radicals by moisturizing and hydrating your skin.

How to do it:

a.   Separate the yolk from an egg carefully

b.   Apply the egg white evenly on clean face

c.   Wait for 15 until it dries and wash it off

5.   Banana

After your menopause, skin problems become your major problem. Luckily, there is a cheap and healthy natural remedy, such as banana, that can treat this problem. Being rich in vitamin E, C, B, and potassium, this fruit will give you supple, elastic, beautiful and healthy skin. It fights any effect of oxidative stress and free radicals by improving collagen production and moisturizing your skin.

How to do it:

a.   Mash two ripe bananas

b.   Apply the paste on clean face

c.   Wait for 30 minutes, then wash it off before applying moisturizer

6. Honey

Honey is your menopause and premature aging solution. With the help of potassium and vitamin B, it prevents your skin from losing its suppleness and elasticity by hydrating the tissue. Besides, it also regenerates new cells, fixes the broken ones, and removes the dead cells to lighten any age spot, scar, and hyper skin pigmentation.

How to do it:

a. Take a teaspoon of honey and put it on your palm

b. Apply the honey gently on clean face with circular motion

c. Wait for 20 minutes and wash it off

7. Lemon juice

Lemon juice is a perfect natural remedy with bleaching property to remove sunburn and tan. It is also quite useful in removing dead cells, exfoliating skin, shrinking open pores, tightening skin tissues, increasing skin elasticity, reducing fine lines and wrinkles, and improving skin complexion. In simple words, you can get your smooth, young, and healthy skin with the help of lemon juice.

How to do it:

a. Take one lemon and squeeze out the juice.

b. Use a cotton ball to dab the juice on clean face.

    c.   Wait for 30 minutes, and then wash it off.

8.   Pineapples

After your menopause, you may also suffer from digestive disorders and pineapple is just a great natural solution for this problem. With high antioxidant contents, such as vitamin C and potassium, pineapple can help you fighting the harmful effects of oxidative stress of cells and free radicals. Other benefits include improved skin tone, brighter skin tone, removed dark patches, less age spots, and reduced hyper pigmentation.

How to do it:

a.   Take ½ cup of pineapple pulp

b.   Use a blender to crush the pulp to make smooth paste

c.   Apply the paste on clean neck and face

d.   Wait for 20 minutes, then wash it off

pH Balance and Aging

Before you decide to take natural remedies to fight premature aging and other post-menopause syndromes, your body will maintain your normal pH balance as the first line of defense against this women's nightmare. It is only when your body has reached the balance between alkaline and acid; you can remain healthy even after menopause.

The more acidic your body, the more effort it will put to restore the acidic-alkaline balance, which is not a good news for your health. Our body will extract calcium from its deposits in our bones, tissue, and teeth. Initial damage would be osteoporosis, teeth damage, and tissue damage. These are the three common post-menopause symptoms. At the same time, taking calcium from its deposits may also increase the pOH (alkaline pH) level and decrease the body pH level.

Understanding the ideal pH-pOH level in our body is the first thing we should do before we fight against premature aging and menopause symptoms. On the pH scale, we use a range of number from one to 14 to express the alkalinity and acidity of a specific substance. While level 1 expresses the highest level (most acidic), level seven expresses the balanced state between alkaline and acid. At the end of the scale, we have level 14, which express the lowest level or the most alkaline one.

Experts measure the ideal pH level for our body from our blood, which is 7.43. In other words, our body is naturally more alkaline than water (pH 7). Any change to this state would mean there is something wrong inside our body. Any pH reading above 7.5 would tell us that our body is running on alkalosis state (overly alkaline state), while any reading under seven would prove the evidence of acidosis (overly acidic state).

Even the slightest change in our pH level may bring more harm than good to our body. When our body starts to experience the overly acidic state, you must prepare yourself to experience these symptoms:

- ✓ Chronic fatigue
- ✓ Difficult weight loss
- ✓ Chronic aches
- ✓ Constipation
- ✓ Skin problems
- ✓ Frequent colds
- ✓ Weak kidneys
- ✓ Sudden weight gain
- ✓ Excessive stress
- ✓ Malaise
- ✓ Headaches
- ✓ Mental confusion

There is one bad news about this pH balance: it happens at hormonal level. It means we will never know when the imbalance begins. We will only know if the pH imbalance has affected our body, which begins with the acid reflux problem.

Acid reflux is a digestive problem when we experience a burning sensation after our stomach acid flows up and reach our throat. This burning sensation indicates our blood has become too acidic and restoring the pH balance is the only way to relieve this problem. During acid reflux, our body is starting to lose its ability to detoxify itself. Without prompt treatment, acid reflux may just be the beginning of other serious illnesses, such as osteoporosis, arthritis, cardiovascular disease, and diabetes.

Reducing acid level throughout our body can help re-balance our blood pH level and heal the digestive tract. We can do this by carefully selecting our foods and beverages. Instead of choosing only foods and beverages we like, we are looking for foods and beverages, which tend to be alkaline to put in our diet. These foods are just the beginning of our mission in restoring our body pH balance.

Our body is no longer as healthy as young women's after our menopause and without a healthy diet, there is no way we can preserve our body and stay as young and healthy as the youth. No matter how difficult and less comfortable the experience, changing our diet is the key towards preventing premature aging. When it comes to pH balancing, fill your diet with alkaline-based meals and avoid processed and manufactured foods, which are usually high in saturated fat.

I also recommend you to follow these tips to balance your body pH:

✓ Manage your stress

✓ Make sure your diet contains 80% alkaline foods and 20% acid-forming foods.

✓ Consume only organic foods

✓ Take vitamins, minerals, and calcium supplements

✓ Cleanse your colon using natural agent regularly, at least every 6 – 12 months.

✓ Drink 8 glasses of water or more every day (not only it will help you balance your blood pH level, but also it will help you hydrate your body)

Besides the above tips, the combination of green raw foods, water, and vegetable juice can also help you regain the pH balance. Taking enough of this healthy foods and beverages combination can improve your digestive tract and reduce your blood acid toxicity.

Based on their acidity levels, we can classify all foods into four main groups. You should make sure you have looked at the following table before placing any meal into your diet:

Food Group	Acidity Rating
Vegetables and Fruits	Alkaline
Eggs and Dairy Products	Acidic
Gravies and Cereals	Acidic
Meats, Fish, and Poultry	Very Acidic

Please note that if you cannot find your meal in the table, I strongly recommend you to consult with your doctor before placing the meal in your diet. A precaution is highly necessary in healthy life.

Doing nothing and keeping the acidosis state in your body will only accelerate the premature aging. It will be similar with choosing to refuse to stay young and healthy after your menopause. If this is your choice, then there is no reason you should continue reading this eBook.

All the sacrifices you made in changing your diet and managing your stress will result in one obvious thing. You will soon experience the dream every woman has after menopause: a healthy life with better metabolism, less external/internal signs of aging, and vitality that is more natural. You may age 50, but your body will stay as young and healthy as you were in your 20. This is your dream and you have done many things so far to achieve it. If there is something better than achieving your dream, then you can leave this healthy lifestyle after your menopause.

44

Ways to Look 10 Years Younger Fast!
*The best way out is always
through.*

--Robert Frost

Reverse any sign of premature aging after your menopause and look a decade younger with these amazing solutions:

1. Eat iron-rich diet

    Iron deficiency is a common cause for dark circles and bags under your eyes. Eating iron-rich diet, such as kidney beans, dark chocolate, and spinach can help you stay young and healthy.

2. Eye primer for beautiful eyes

    Your makeup can settle into crevices and wrinkles if you apply it on your eyelids, giving them a prominent state. Use an eye primer to counter the effect and your makeup will go as smooth and long as you want.

3. Your eyebrows need touch

    Do not over pluck your eyebrows. As when we reached 40, over tweezing our eye brows will only make us look like losing this beautiful part of our face, not to mention it is also a classic sign of premature aging and menopause.

4.   Moisturize your skin

If you want youthful-looking eyes, please do not forget to moisturize your skin as dry skin usually leads to bags, wrinkles, and cracks. If you are having problem with puffiness, a calendula eye balm or gel eye serum may provide the answer. You may also opt for a nighttime retinol cream if your crow's feet disturb you.

5.   Keep salt away

Consuming too much salt may result in water retention in your eyes. As I believe you hate having this problem after your menopause, try to limit your salt intake up to 2,300 milligrams or around 1 teaspoon a day.

6.   Sweet potato eye pads

You do not need to go to a spa to get the spa-grade eye pad. Instead of using cucumbers, you can switch them with sweet potatoes. With their anti-inflammatory properties and dense mass, you can use them to reduce that puffiness.

How to do it:

Take each potato and cut into 1-inch slices. In the morning, place the slices on both eyes and wait for 10 minutes for it to reduce puffiness and darkness.

7. Grab different eye liner

    You are doing it wrong if you think wearing dark eyeliner on the bottom and top lash line would give you the perfect look. Instead, it will only darken the dark circles and draw the crow's feet. For this reason, I recommend you to only use the dark eyeliner above your top lash line and use another light eyeliner to line the bottom lash line. You can also brighten your look by using a light shadow on your creases.

8. Brussel sprouts and olive oil are preferable

    Brussels sprouts and olive oil has been quite famous for their anti-aging properties. Using these natural remedies, you can keep your eyes healthy, prevent them from cataracts and vision loss as well as any age-related eye macular degeneration.

9. Enjoy your green tea

    Use tea bags to fight your eye bags! Freeze your green tea pouches for a while, and then rest them on your eyes to reduce puffiness. The tanine substance inside the pouch will help reduce blood swelling and constrict your blood vessels.

10.   Lighten dark circles

There is no such thing as miracle product that can eliminate your under-eye circles instantly. Instead of wasting your money, you can use concealer to lighten your under-eye bags. A creamy concealer should be able to help you, especially the one with yellow undertones, as it will neutralize any purple hue.

Look Younger with Make Up, New Hairstyle, a More Youthful Smile, New Wardrobe

Success is the sum of small efforts, repeated day in and day out.

--Robert Collier

It has always been in our DNA: as women, we would love to live a healthy and beautiful life. We have done everything we could, but as we age, our body experiences a rapid hormonal decrease. We are losing our body functions. Our cells, tissues, organs, and muscles are not working as good as 10 – 20 years ago. This degenerative function becomes worse as we reache menopause. Our skin is losing its beauty, suppleness, and elasticity. The first good news is that we can slow down the degenerative process by living a healthy lifestyle. The next good news is that we can still preserve our beauty, but only if we follow these simple makeup tips that will make us look younger almost instantly.

1. Choose lighter lipstick

   After our menopause, our lips get thinner. This is not good, as dark shades may not appear as beautiful as we expect. To prevent lipstick from becoming another nightmare after our menopause, use flesh-colored or rosy-red shades as your lipstick color. Keep away from oranges and peaches, as your teeth may appear yellow with this color around.

2. Your apples need special touch

   Makeup can lift your cheek instantly. First, make sure you have placed your blush brush at the top of your cheekbone, and then apply your favorite color gently in circular motion. For the best look, you can choose bronzes, apricots, or pinks.

3. Use pencil to lift your eyes

   Instead of using liquid liners, you can use the softness of your eye pencil to enlarge your eyes. Avoid the droopy-looking lids by blending the liner up at your eyes outer corners using the Q-tip.

4. You need an extra-large sunglasses

   At the previous chapter of this eBook, I have told you how harmful our sun can be. Therefore, besides using sunblock to moisture your skin, why do not you try using fashionable sunglasses? Well, not only it makes you look fashionable, but also it can protect your eyes. I recommend using the oversize frames rather than the thinly rimmed aviators for extra protection area around your beautiful eyes. You can also use a scarf to prevent sunspots on your skin.

5. Moisturize your hands

    After our menopause, our skin is getting easier to dry and lose its suppleness, elasticity, and beauty. In order to keep your hands youthful looking, apply a retinoid-rich product on your hands. This product should be the same with the one you use on your face. Then, you can add an extra layer of Vaseline. To keep the treatment intact, you can also wear cotton gloves while sleeping. Within few days, you can feel your skin turn supple and smooth again.

6. Love your feet

    Dry and rough feet are the last thing any woman should have. They make us look older, no matter shoes we wear. Treating our feet is the first thing we should do to get those sexy and beautiful feet back again. Before wearing shoes, apply salicylic acid on your feet, but remember to keep it thin. Then, you can apply a dollop of your moisturizer to certain areas where you get scaly or thick skin. Once you have applied it, you can wear your socks.

This short treatment will keep your feet beautiful by keeping the blisters and calluses away.

7. Grab yourself a self-tanner

A self-tanner can heal your skin and bring back its beauty, but you need to use it carefully as excessive use may also emphasize and even darken your sunspots. If you experience any damage due to the self-tanner, you can apply a warm foundation shade, which will slowly reverse the effect.

8. Eliminate brown spots

Sunspots are undoubtedly one of the most irritating skin problems. Luckily, you just need to dilute a glass of lemon juice with water to fade these irritating spots, no matter what skin tone you have. Please remember that lemon juice might be irritating. Therefore, I recommend you to applying it using a Q-tip before going to bed. Gradually increase the treatment to twice daily and stop it after you have your dream skin, without being too light.

9. Antioxidant-infused sunscreens for your skin

SPF 30 is necessary for a beautiful skin, but it is not the only skin protection we have. An antioxidant-infused sunscreen can also protect your skin by reducing the oxidative damage due to the sun exposure. However, please do not apply this sunscreen often as they trigger inflammatory problems.

10. Remove your makeup before night rest

There are two main reasons you should remove your makeup before going to bed. First, it helps you prevent clogged pores. Second, it is highly likely there are harmful agents inside your makeup after whole-day exposure to polluted environment. Washing away your makeup will eliminate these agents, prevent collagen breakdown, and keep your skin elastic.

FAQ

The following section contains questions women asked about their life after menopause. In this section, you can find almost everything you want to know about your life after menopause.

1.   Will my voice change after menopause?

Most women do not experience this concern after their menopause; however, some women may still become subject of this change.

2.   I am experiencing facial hair growth few months after my menopause. Is there something I can do about this?

There are only few medical reports when women experience facial hair growth after their menopause. However, this concern may still become troublesome for some women. If you experience this problem, you can opt for depilatories (using creams or liquids to remove facial hair), waxing, prescription cream, bleaching, laser hair removal, and electrolysis. Please consult with your doctor to determine the best facial hair treatment for you.

3. Is it true that once women entered their menopause, they should still concern about birth control?

    If your last period was a year ago, this is a clear evidence that you have entered your menopause. Until you are certain of this evidence, I strongly recommend you to continuing your birth control program if you use any.

4. Is it normal when my hot flushes are not as frequent as I heard from one of my friends?

    Hot flushes or flashes are common symptoms during perimenopause. However, not all women experience this symptom and not all flushes come with the same frequency. You may experience mild hot flushes, while your friend might experience hot flashes severe enough to disrupt her sleep. There are also some cases when women experience night sweats during their perimenopause. It is also a common occurrence for hot flushes to last for 30 – 60 seconds, but in some cases, they may continue for years or even decades.

5.   I am at my premenopausal stage and my doctor told me to take birth control pills at low dose. May I know the reason?

If you are currently at premenopausal stage, your doctor might recommend you to taking low-dose birth control pills for safety precaution. With only 20 micrograms of estrogen, these pills are safe enough before you entered your final period.

6.   How I benefit from taking birth control pills at low dose?

There are certain benefits low-dose birth control pills can give you. First, it can help you prevent pregnancy. Second, it can regular irregular or even heavy menstrual periods. Third, it protects your body against uterine and ovarian cancer as well as osteoporosis.

7.   Is there any other way I can treat my hot flushes, besides the hormone replacement therapy?

Hormone Replacement Therapy (HRT) is the most recommended hot flashes treatment as it delivers the best result. However, you may also opt for other treatments that share the same purpose. However, please consult with your doctor before choosing any of these alternative treatments. Alternative hot flushes treatments include:

- ✓ Low-dose paroxetine, venlafaxine, or fluoxetine (depression drugs)
- ✓ Clonidine (blood pressure medication)
- ✓ Brisdelle
- ✓ Duavee
- ✓ Gabapentin

8. Should I worry about hormone replacement therapy?

As with all medicines, Hormone Replacement Therapy contains both benefits and risks. From a Women's Health Initiative study, there is a clear evidence that when a therapy combines progesterone and estrogen treatment, it possess long-term risk of increased risk of blood clots, breast cancer, stroke, and heart disease. The same study also revealed that why estrogen is not accountable for the increasing risk of heart disease or breast cancer, any therapy that involves estrogen as a single agent might increase the risk of stroke and blood clots.

Using the data Women's Health Initiative provided, the US government through the US Preventative Services Task Force decided not to recommend performing Hormone Replacement Therapy to treat or prevent chronic diseases, including, but not limited to heart disease, dementia, and osteoporosis. Even though this treatment still offer benefits to cure the illness, the risks are still greater than the benefits. If you experience any of these benefits after your menopause and considering taking HRT, please consult with your doctor to find the best treatment available for you.

9. Is there any alternative treatment I can take to treat my menopause symptoms?

If you choose natural remedies for your menopause, you can try consuming botanical supplements with high level of estrogen-like substances, such as soy. These natural remedies may relieve your menopausal symptoms. If you are experiencing hot flushes or night sweats after your menopause, you can also try some black cohoshes, which may relieve you from the less comfortable experience. These natural remedies may offer other benefits for your menopausal treatment, but they may also contain risks. Therefore, further medical studies are necessary to weigh any risk and benefit regarding these natural remedies. It would act as a good prevention if you consult with your doctor before taking any natural remedy to relieve your menopausal symptom.

10.   I no longer enjoy having sex since my menopause. How can I fix this?

After your menopause, you may experience pain while having sex. Please do not panic as this pain occurs to most women after their menopause. Your body is losing its estrogen due to the menopause. Estrogen is an important hormone that keeps your vaginal tissue thick enough for sexual activity. When there is not enough estrogen in your body, you will experience vaginal dryness. However, there might be another aspect that cause the pain. Try to visit your doctor and discuss about this to find out all possible causes.

Some people may recommend you taking lubricants to relieve the pain. As temporary treatment, it may work. To find which lubricant fits you the most, please ask your pharmacist or doctor. When necessary, your doctor may also recommend you to taking one or more local estrogen treatments, such as estrogen ring, cream, or tablets to 'moisturize' your vagina.

Only with medical prescription, you can also take Osphena, an oral drug for menopausal symptom, once a day. This medication will thicken your vaginal tissue, making it less fragile. As the result, you will experience less pain while having sex.

If you enjoyed this book or found it useful in some way, I would like to ask you for a favor. Would you be kind enough **to leave a review** for this book? It would be appreciated greatly!

Thank you very much.

Dominique Kaneza, Author

Join the exclusive mailing list to get updates and free books

www.tmapublishing.com